T0250393

WHAT IS PSYCHOANALYSIS?

Founded by C. K. Ogden

The International Library of Psychology

PSYCHOANALYSIS
In 28 Volumes

WHAT IS PSYCHOANALYSIS?

ISADOR H CORIAT

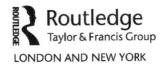

LONDON AND NEW YORK

First published in 1919 by
Routledge, Trench, Trubner & Co., Ltd.
2 Park Square, Milton Park, Abingdon, Oxfordshire OX14 4RN
711 Third Avenue, New York, NY 10017

First issued in paperback 2014

Routledge is an imprint of the Taylor and Francis Group, an informa business

British Library Cataloguing in Publication Data
A CIP catalogue record for this book
is available from the British Library

What Is Psychoanalysis?
ISBN 0415-21086-0
Psychoanalysis: 28 Volumes
ISBN 0415-21132-8
The International Library of Psychology: 204 Volumes
ISBN 0415-19132-7

ISBN 13: 978-1-138-87555-5 (pbk)
ISBN 13: 978-0-415-21086-7 (hbk)

INTRODUCTION

The origin and purpose of this book may be stated in a few words. From time to time physicians, clergymen, social workers, and laymen have made certain enquiries concerning psychoanalysis, with particular reference to its aim and purpose and its field of usefulness as a therapeutic procedure. These questions were recorded and the answers planned, partly on the basis of the theory of psychoanalysis, and partly with a view to meeting certain objections and criticisms which were made at the time the questions were answered. Much of these data is incorporated in the present little volume.

The answers to these questions, while explaining psychoanalysis, have at the same time provided suggestions for mental hygiene and character formation. It is hoped that this volume will answer satisfactorily the various enquiries which puzzle people in a scientific field so new and epoch-making and so little understood as that of psychoanalysis. The nature of the book renders a little repetition necessary and unavoidable.

The neuroses are the most distressing and frequent of human ills, and to a greater degree than physical diseases; they lead to social inefficiency. In severe bodily disorders, the patient can utilise his inner resources for compensation and consolation, but in the neuroses he is robbed of these resources, since the mind is torn by emotional conflicts. It is here that psychoanalysis is most efficacious, because it brings relief from within, from the inner resources of the sufferer. Psychoanalysis is recognised to-day as the most important advance in methods of a rational and scientific psychotherapy. It is applicable to all nervous disorders of mental origin which make up so large a part of the practice of medicine.

This volume does not profess to teach psychoanalysis, as this can be learned only by long training and study by one already experienced in nervous and mental diseases. The character of the book permits only a minimum of theory and discussion. A brief bibliography is appended for those who may wish further information on the subject.

ISADOR H. CORIAT.

CONTENTS

WHAT IS PSYCHOANALYSIS?

ARRANGED IN QUESTIONS AND ANSWERS

Q. What is psychoanalysis?

A. Psychoanalysis is the most recent and advanced therapeutic procedure for the treatment of the neuroses. It is what its name implies, an analysis of the mind. Other psychotherapeutic methods deal only with the superficial manifestations of the neuroses, and therefore cannot produce a fundamental cure. Psychoanalysis concerns itself primarily with the cause of symptoms, with their real underlying mechanism. It not only penetrates into the origin of symptoms, but the analysis at the same time is the treatment.

It is a study of man's unconscious motives

and desires as shown in various nervous disturbances and in certain mainifestations of every-day life in normal individuals. It has been demonstrated that the manifold symptoms of the neuroses result from unfulfilled desires, often extending back to the earliest years of childhood. These desires not only influence the formation of character traits, but likewise are responsible for many forms of nervous illness.

Q. Where and under what conditions did psychoanalysis originate ?

A. The evolution of psychoanalysis forms an interesting chapter in the history of medicine. It was in 1881 that Freud, in association with Breuer of Vienna, whose name is well known for his researches on the physiology of the semicircular canals, started to treat a young woman who was suffering from hysteria. The usual means were tried in vain, until it was found that the facts offered by the patient in explanation of her condition represented only a part of the history. This was not due to a deliberate attempt on the part of the patient to conceal her medical antecedents, but as it later developed, to an unconscious repression, because the emotional state which was a part of these concealed facts represented painful experiences. Finally by a procedure, which later developed into the refinements of the psychoanalytic method, many hidden experiences of the past with their attached emotions were brought to light, and it was shown that it was these experiences which caused the hysterical condition. These memories, although buried in the unconscious, were active and living forces, and only when they were lived over again did a cure take place. They were not merely forgotten but repressed, although unconsciously so, and it was only when this repression was overcome that the patient began to improve.

At first hypnosis was employed to revive the forgotten memories, but later it was discovered that hypnosis was not necessary in psychoanalysis, and since then its use has been abandoned. In 1895 Breuer and Freud published their studies on the mechanism of hysteria, in which it was shown that the hysterical symptoms arose from reminiscences unknown to and forgotten by the sufferer. They demonstrated that the forgetting was a purposeful act, in the same way that a normal individual conveniently " forgets " the unpleasant experiences of his life.

In 1900, Freud published his great work on the " Interpretation of Dreams," and there was opened up a new field of investigation of the unconscious in both normal and abnormal conditions. Nervous patients frequently related strange dreams to him and it was found that each dream possessed a profound personal significance for the dreamer, in fact, it was the outgrowth, sometimes literal, sometimes symbolic, of the individual's unconscious mental life. It was definitely proven that every dream was the fulfilment of repressed wishes. Dream analysis revealed the mechanism of delusions, morbid fears, hysteria, fixed ideas and compulsive thinking, and at the same time it provided neurology the most potent instrument for the removal of these abnormal symptoms in the form of what became known as the psychoanalytic treatment.

Thus the fundamental and basic idea of Freud's work is that a large number of normal and abnormal mental processes come from hidden sources, unknown and unsuspected by the individual. The gulf between normal thinking and abnormal mental states has been definitely bridged by psychoanalysis, for instance, when it is stated, that the normal " forgetting " of an unpleasant experience is identical but to a more limited degree, with the repressions of an hysteric.

Q. To what other fields of investigation has psychoanalysis been applied besides that of medicine ?

A. Psychoanalysis has entered many new fields of thought. These various principles of Freud's psychology and the psychoanalytic method have been successfully applied in not only helping the nervously ill, but the same fundamental principles have been used to interpret the unconscious sources of wit, literary creations, myths, folk lore and the slips of the tongue and forgetting of normal individuals. It was demonstrated that the unconscious mental processes which formed dreams were identical with those at work in imaginative creations in literature, in wit, in the social consciousness and in that folk spirit from which myths and folk lore are elaborated.

Psychoanalysis is beginning to found a new ethics as well as a new psychology, a new neurology and a new school of literary criticism.   It bears the same relation in all its principles to the human mind, and to the social consciousness, as biology does to the organic world.

Freud's principal works are his papers on hysteria and the psychoneuroses, the three contributions to the sexual theory, the work on interpretation of dreams,* the psycho-pathology of everyday life, the monograph entitled " Totem and Taboo," the psycho-analytic study of Leonardo da Vinci and finally the contribution on wit and its rela-tion to the unconscious.

* See the answer to the question on the origin of psycho-analysis.

In his three contributions to the sexual theory, Freud deals principally with the development of the sexual instinct in its relationship to repression, both social and individual, and the part played by repression in the evolution of abnormal mental states.

In the psychopathology of everyday life it is shown that the unconscious mental mechanism which produces errors in writing and speech, the forgetting of familiar names and words, slips of tongue and the like, is identical with the mental mechanism which produces the psychoneuroses.

The work on "Totem and Taboo" is devoted to demonstrating that the individual and social defence reactions and the symbolisation of repressed feelings is the same in savage man as in the educated individual, that is, the taboos of a primitive group are essentially identical with the taboos of civilised society.

The study of Leonardo da Vinci is based

upon a fragment of one of Leonardo's infantile memories and, by a most ingenious logic, this fragment is utilised to explain Leonardo's greatness as an artist and man of science and to fathom the mystery of the smile of Mona Lisa.

In the book on wit is shown that wit and laughter are merely methods through which the unconscious obtains the greatest amount of pleasure within the shortest space of time, and that the psychological structure of a joke very much resembles the psychological structure of a dream.

In addition to Freud, other investigators have published valuable studies and investigations on the various medical and cultural aspects of psychoanalysis, such as the relation between myths and dreams, comparative mythology, sketches of great artists and finally psychoanalytic interpretations of complex literary creations, such as Hamlet and Lady Macbeth.

Q. To whom should the practice of psychoanalysis be limited ?

A. To those thoroughly trained in the theory of psychoanalysis and in general psychopathology. For an untrained person to use psychoanalysis is as much to be deprecated as it is for some one to use radium who is ignorant of the physics of radio-activity, or as dangerous as to attempt a surgical operation without a knowledge of anatomy.

Q. What is the attitude of physicians trained in nervous and mental diseases towards psychoanalysis ?

A. Some are sympathetic, other antagonise the psychoanalytic movement. On reading the criticisms of psychoanalysis, however, it will be found that they are chiefly remarkable for their complete misapprehension of the theories and purposes of psychoanalysis. There is a refusal to make an honest examination of the subject. The chief misunderstandings are along the lines of the sexual etiology of the neuroses, the manner in which psychoanalysis works, transference,* and the technical methods of dream analysis and interpretation.

Q. Can psychoanalysis be harmful ?

A. " Wild " psychoanalysis is a term first introduced by Freud and refers to the gross errors into which some physicians fall who have a hazy idea of the principles and teachings of psychoanalysis and attempt to apply them in their practice. The serious errors which may take place are incorrect advice concerning sexual difficulties, an over-emphasis on the part of the psycho-analyst on sexual matters, when these are

* Explained in the answer to the question on transference.

shown merely as symbols in the dreams or symptoms of the neurosis and the improper utilisation of the transference. Furthermore, the mental factor in the neuroses must not be overlooked, neither must the analyst fall into the error that it is the ignorance of sexual matters which needs enlightenment and which are producing the neurosis. In addition, in the sexual neuroses, such as homo-sexuality, the advice which is usually given concerning attempts at sexual indulgence, is to be strongly condemned, partly for moral reasons and partly for the fact that the patient does not need such advice as he is fully aware of his difficulties. The analysis must be non-personal, the physician must be the scientist. During the course of the analysis, the reading of psychoanalytic literature must be strongly advised against, since such reading may produce a mental attitude which becomes a strong resistance.

Q. What is the cause of certain failures in psychoanalysis ?

A. Failures in psychoanalysis are due either to bad technique, the lack of transference, the strength of resistance* and finally to the type of case which the physician is attempting to treat. If the technique is at fault, the physician is unable to interpret or root out the unconscious factors of the neurosis, or he may be unable to handle the transference or resistances as they should be handled. In those cases which do not progress to recovery after treatment has been carried out for a sufficiently long period, it will be found that the failure is due either to—

1. Impossibility of a complete transference.

2. The development of resistance due to

---

* Both this term and also " transference," which are so important for psychoanalysis, are explained in the answers to the questions dealing with these subjects.

some present situation or to a mooring to infantile factors.

3. Inability to break down the disturbing unconscious complexes.

4. A desire on the part of the patient to retain the neurosis, since the neurosis acts as a withdrawal from a reality which was found to be unbearable. In other words, under these conditions, paradoxical as it may seem, the nervous illness is preferred to mental health, since the nervous illness acts as a sort of a protector.

5. In imperfectly selected cases, since psychoanalysis should not be used in delirious states, in persons over fifty years of age, since their nervous systems lack a certain plasticity, in cases of acute hysteria or in severe mental diseases.

Q. Has psychoanalysis definite laws ?

A. Yes, as definite as the laws of gravitation, even though it deals with mental instead of physical phenomena. Psychoanalysis is both scientific and technical and from its data there has developed a new science. It has nothing to do with the ordinary history of the nervous illness as given by the patient, for the latter tells his physician only his conscious thoughts, which are revealed either as replies to direct questions or as a spontaneous recital of the difficulties. Patients too frequently attribute their nervous illness to circumstances which act merely as precipitating causes and bear no relation to the real underlying motive of the illness. The most frequent of these misconceptions is attributing their neurosis to overwork. It is the reduction of these conscious contents of the mind through certain well recognised and elaborated technical methods, to their real unconscious sources in the matters of cause and effect, with which psychoanalysis primarily deals.

Psychoanalysis presupposes that there is no mental effect without its cause, and consequently nervous symptoms are not chance and haphazard products, but are related to definite mental processes which are repressed in the patient's unconscious. This relation of mental cause and effect is called determinism. By means of the study of dreams and symptomatic actions, and sometimes by use of the association tests, psychoanalysis traces out each symptom in the patient's life history. Sometimes these symptoms are found to be deeply buried in the earliest years of childhood. It handles what are known as the patient's emotional transferences, finds out the cause for any resistance to the analysis, and finally guides the patient to a utilisation of his energy along more useful social lines than that of the neurotic conflict. All this requires the expert trained in the theoretical and practical aspects of psychoanalysis.

Q. Does psychoanalysis apply to the abnormal only ?

A. No, it also gives an insight into the workings of normal minds and it may assist in changing certain detrimental character traits in those who are actually not nervously ill.

Q. Have the methods of psychoanalysis been proven practically and theoretically ?

A. Entirely so, since the practical results in the cure of cases of severe nervous illness completely harmonises with the theories which lie at the basis of psychoanalysis.

Q. What types of cases are most suitable for psychoanalysis ?

A. The cases to which psychoanalysis is applicable and in which its best results are recorded, consist principally of the severe hysterias, the compulsion neuroses and anxiety neuroses (formerly grouped under the term of psychasthenia), stammering, neurasthenia, sexual neurasthenia, the sexual neuroses (sadism, masochism, homo-sexuality, psychical impotence, etc.), and finally certain psychoses, such as mild cases of manic-depressive insanity, and in the early stages of dementia præcox and para-noiac states. Psychoanalysis may also be of help in cases of kleptomania and in determining the underlying motives in certain cases of juvenile delinquency, when these are uncomplicated by mental defect or feeble mindedness.

Q. What class of patients are most diffi-cult to treat by psychoanalysis ?

A. Persons over fifty, cases of severe stammering and cases of far advanced.

paranoia or dementia præcox. A sceptical attitude is no obstacle to a successful psychoanalysis since this scepticism is a form of resistance which can easily be overcome.

Q. Does psychoanalysis tend to produce an unhealthy introspection ?

A. On the contrary, its methods are directly opposed to those of introspection.

Q. How does psychoanalysis differ from mere introspection ?

A. Introspection merely records the superficial facts of consciousness. It makes no attempt to trace the cause of our various ideas, neither does it examine the unconscious contents and motives of the human mind.

Q. Is psychoanalysis a kind of confession ?

A. A great relief may be gained by a secular confession and yet the confession of a repressed idea of a secret mental anguish does not cure, and if improvement takes place, it is only temporary. This fact in itself invalidates the idea that the beneficial effect of psychoanalysis is through free unburdening and mental catharsis. Psychoanalysis works through transference, the overcoming of resistances, its ability to penetrate into the unconscious and not to a free confession.

Q. Does not the element of suggestion enter into psychoanalysis; that is, the patient's belief or faith that the method employed will cure him?

A. Under no circumstances. If psychoanalysis is carried out in the manner it should be, no explanations or suggestions are made to the patient during the course of treatment. Gradually the patient begins to see things for himself, begins to understand his inner life, and actually starts to get well or even be cured before he grasps the real significance of the psychoanalytic procedure. Furthermore, a large percentage of patients undertake the psychoanalytic treatment with a great deal of scepticism, as they have become profoundly discouraged from their previous attempts to get well. Psychoanalysis helps, not because of explanations or suggestion, but because it teaches a policy of non-resistance towards the neurosis and takes the responsibility (transference) of the cure. Non-resistance is the first step in a psychoanalysis.

Q. How does psychoanalysis differ from suggestion?

A. Those who have first used suggestive methods and later substituted psychoanalysis for them, have seen the immeasurable superiority of the latter over the former. Psychoanalysis reaches the fundamental difficulties of the nervous illness, whereas suggestion merely side tracks it, or covers it up for the time being. The most important instrument of psychoanalysis is the interpretations of the dreams, as throwing light upon the real unconscious of the nervous sufferer, for it is in the unconscious that the neurosis has taken its origin. Both the dreams and the neurosis originate from the same unconscious sources. The method by which psychoanalysis works is directly opposite to the usual psychotherapeutic procedures of hypnosis, persuasion and suggestion.

Freud has emphasised the difference between psychoanalysis and suggestion, by pointing out that the former takes something away, that is the power which the abnormal mental processes have over the patient, while the latter puts something on, in adding the force of the suggestion in opposition to that of the neurosis. In the most efficacious method of suggestion, that is hypnosis, it is well known that it is practically impossible to hypnotise certain people, while every one can be psychoanalysed. Psychoanalysis does not force anything upon the patient which the latter does not see for himself and which meets with his understanding. Psychoanalysis brings self knowledge, although this self knowledge is not acquired without a struggle.

Q. Is the cure wholly due to psychoanalysis, or to other factors such as those who manage to get on their feet from work, suggestion, encouragement or the advice of the physician ?

A. The cure is wholly due to psychoanalysis, since when patients get well through other methods, the neurosis is likely to break out again at some critical emotional period. Psychoanalysis removes the cause of the symptoms, other methods merely change the mental attitude towards symptoms which still persist or at the best, they remove only the surface manifestations.

Q. How does psychoanalysis work ?

A. Principally through transference. The analysis attracts to itself the emotions which are set free in the course of the analysis. These emotions are then changed by the analytic process, to a new and more useful form of energy. In the analysis, the physician plays the part of the impersonal agent which has the specific effect of splitting off the energy attached to the repressed ideas causing the neurosis and using this energy for the purpose of a cure. Psychoanalysis enables the patient to utilise his reserve energy for a better purpose than that of struggling with the nervous illness.

Q. What is transference ?

A. Transference is not only the central problem of psychoanalyis, but it is the most difficult and delicate problem to handle. All psychoanalysis proceeds through what is called " transference " and it is in the method of handling the transferences, that constitutes the great superiority of psycho-analysis in treating the neuroses. Trans-ference may be defined as a feeling of acknowledged sympathy from the patient to the physician; the same occurs in all lines of medical treatment when the patient has confidence in his physician. In neurotic patients this feeling is much more exagger-ated and therefore the sympathetic relation to the physician becomes more intense than in patients with organic disease.

Transference is therefore not a specific

35

result of psychoanalytic treatment, neither is transference limited to psychoanalysis, but it appears here much more clearly, since neurotics have a deeper craving for sympathy than those who are not nervously ill. In psychoanalytic treatment, the transference must be delicately handled and not at all abused ; in fact, the object of the physician is to release the patient from the transferences which have developed during the course of the analysis and break them up. It is the handling of the transferences which makes psychoanalysis so difficult, because one must be careful that the effect of this transference between physician and patient does not become permanent, namely, the dependence on the physician must be cut off. In other words, the patient at the end of the treatment and when he is cured, must be left an independent personality. Every successful analysis does this. Transference is a barometer of the patient's feelings towards the physician and towards the neurosis. All conflicts must be fought out in the territory of transference.

The ethical value of psychoanalysis depends upon telling a patient the truth and maintaining a perfectly sincere attitude. The patient must not drive away the transference or retain it, but both patient and physician must treat it as a temporary manifestation occurring during the period of treatment. A neurotic's interests are turned within himself ; he cannot be made efficient until his interests are projected outside on the practical affairs of life. Transference must be handled delicately and scientifically, in the same way that a chemist handles explosives or a surgeon cuts into delicate nerve tissues.

Q. How does the transference show itself ?

A. In the reactions of the patient, in dreams, and in the rapidity by which the symptoms of the nervous illness subside and disappear.

Q. What is resistance ?

A. Resistance is the opposite of transference. It is the substitution of a hostile feeling for a sympathetic one. Resistance may have several sources and, like transference, is really derived from the patient's unconscious. Resistance arises during the unconscious battle of intellect and instinct, which is going on in every neurotic. It is the force exerted which prevents unwelcome and unpleasant thoughts from becoming conscious. This process is particularly well seen in dreams because what is termed the " censor " in dreams, attempts to prevent all the dream thoughts from coming out in an analysis, as so many of these thoughts deal with the deepest recesses of the personality. Resistance is the skeleton in the closet which plays havoc with the peace of mind. The skeleton is the hidden complex, the repressed or secret anguish. The attempt to open the door on this skeleton is often the source of a severe unconscious and even conscious struggle in psychoanalytic treatment. This struggle is the resistance, and no psychoanalysis can be successful until these resistances are broken down, until the opposite of resistance, the transference, is obtained.

Any obstacle which a patient opposes to his recovery is a form of resistance. Resistance, like transference, is often indicated in the dreams. The patient resists getting well, because getting well brings him in touch with reality again, whereas the neurosis, through which he withdraws into himself, offers a refuge from reality. Hence the apparently paradoxical statement of psychoanalysis becomes clear, when it is stated that the patient gains something by his nervous illness and therefore dreads getting well. It is probably this form of resistance, above all other factors, which explains the long duration of nervous illnesses and the difficulty of successfully treating them. In other words, resistance is the effort of the patient to defend his neurosis from disappearing through psychoanalysis. The reading of psychoanalytic literature in some cases may increase the resistance and this kind of self knowledge tends to lengthen rather than shorten the treatment. The resistances of a patient should not be criticised as their sources are unconscious. The breaking down of resistances should be left to the physician and not attempted by the patient. Confidence comes when the resistances are overcome.

Q. What is meant by a complex ?

A. An idea with emotions grouped around it and attached to it, is termed a complex. A complex may consist of painful memories which are banished into the unconscious, but not really forgotten, since such complexes may appear in dreams, symptomatic actions or form the underlying mechanism of a neurosis. This species of forgetting is purposeful, in order to defend the mind from painful memories. Such purposeful forgetting is termed repression. One of the most important of these complexes is termed the Œdipus-complex.

Q. What is the Œdipus-complex ?

A. This complex has its origin during the earliest years of childhood, and consists of an over-attachment of the son to the mother. In certain children as they develop into adulthood, there is a breaking away from these infantile attachments. Other children never break away, they never put aside their childhood feelings and infantile attachments, but carry these throughout life repressed in the unconscious. These children become neurotics, since the repressed complex furnishes the underlying origin of many psychoneuroses and abnormal sexual inversions. It is such a repressed complex which in adults gives rise to dreams of death of one of the parents, usually the opposite parent to that of the infantile attachment. When there is an over-attachment of the daughter to the father, it is termed the Electra-complex. Both terms are taken from Greek mythology, as they are identical with the family situations of two of the greatest Greek tragedies, the Electra of Euripides and the Œdipus Rex of Sophocles. These two complexes lie at the very source of many nervous illnesses. Of course it must be emphasised that these attachments occur more or less intensely in the lives of all children, and it is only when they take an exaggerated form or are not handled properly, that they become a source of danger for the developing child. It is this Œdipus-complex which frequently lies at the basis of homosexuality.

Q. What is homosexuality?

A. This never occurs where the sexual development is normal, hence it is not congenital, but always acquired. It may be defined as an abnormal deviation of the sexual instinct, in which the attachment is for the same instead of for the opposite sex.

Q. How can parents avoid the dangers of over-attachment of their children?

A. The great danger in all these situations, is, that the parents never realise it and the child develops into manhood or womanhood and alone feels or knows the situation. The condition is really an erotic one and hence the large number of individuals who develop homosexuality in adult life. Parents must not allow over-caressing from their children or show an over-exuberant affection for them. The appearance of a new child in the family must not be the signal for the neglect of the other children, as this often leads to secret jealousies.

Q. What is a symptomatic action?

A. This is an action, such as a slip of the tongue or the forgetting of a familiar name, or even a mistake in writing, which is apparently due to chance or excused on the basis of awkwardness. Analysis, however, will demonstrate that the error is of the nature of an unconscious intention. Such symptomatic actions are frequent in the lives of normal people and still more frequently appear in the psychoanalytic treatment of neurotics. In both cases they are produced by unconscious thoughts. A symptomatic action in a normal individual is really a tiny edition of a neurosis, since it has the same unconscious background as a neurosis.

Q. What is repression and how does it produce a neurosis ?

A. Repression is a defence of the mind under normal and abnormal conditions to neutralise or put out of action unwelcome and unpleasant thoughts. These thoughts are pushed back into the unconscious, become repressed and the effort of these repressed thoughts to find an outlet, produces the nervous illness. The mind attempts to find a refuge and free itself from mental conflicts through repression. A great deal of the " forgetting " which occurs in normal individuals and in cases of nervous illness, is not due to any actual decay of memory, as is commonly supposed, but to an active repression. Repression underlies the forgetting of dreams, those losses of memory for limited periods of time termed amnesia, somnambulism and also the condition known as double or multiple personality. The repressed conflict may find an outlet and be expressed in what is known as projection. This projection may manifest itself in peculiar nervous symptoms of a symbolic nature or even as actual delusions, hallucinations, fixed ideas or compulsive thinking. The dream is the most common symbolic representation of repressed thoughts.

Q. How is the term " sexual " used in psychoanalysis ?

A. The term " sex " like " wish " is very broadly used in psychoanalysis. It does not limit itself to referring to the reproductive instinct, neither does it mean that the chief objective of psychoanalysis is to drag out a patient's sexual experiences. Sexual is not the equivalent of sensual, but refers to the fundamental instinct which lies at the very heart of the emotional life, called the libido.

Q. What is meant by the term libido?

A. Libido means vital energy or instinct. It is not always sexual, since the instinct may be hunger or nutritional, beginning as infantile pleasure in nutrition and gradually shading over into the sexual. Thus hunger and sexuality are the two primal human instincts, which are the basis, or to use a technical term, form the root-complex of every neurosis.

Q. What is meant by the " root " of a neurosis?

A. The root of a neurosis is a term used to denote the fundamental unconscious cause of the neurosis, and not the conscious cause as interpreted by the nervous sufferer.

Q. What is the psychoanalytic conception of sexuality ?

A. The child brings his sexual instincts into the world with him. These instincts later may be refined or sublimated into higher forms of energy, or if this does not take place, various perversions and abnormal sexual cravings may develop in the adult. A child's sexuality is first turned on itself ; it is auto-erotic, then it transfers, or fixes itself to those nearest about him and finally, as adult life is reached, it transfers it to a person outside the family group. This last constitutes what is termed falling in love. The sexual components of the child's instincts produce all the neurotic symptoms later in life. It is the unconscious sexual desires and not the conscious sexual ideas which have the strongest influences over us. The word sexual is used in a very wide sense in psychoanalysis. The sexual instinct displays itself very early in the child, first as the sucking or nutritional instinct, secondly as the child grows older, the fixation of its love on the family group or its nurse and thirdly in the sexual changes at puberty.

In this last period, the auto-erotic character of the sexual instinct which characterised infancy and childhood, is lost and a sexual aim is created accompanied by profound physiological changes in the body.

Q. Does psychoanalysis tend to over-emphasise the sexual elements in the neuroses ?

A. Psychoanalysis does not exploit the sexual experiences of patients ; it is not a

4

mere unearthing and exploration of pornographic material. In fact, if psychoanalysis be properly carried out, it refers less to sexual activities than does the usual medical history of an organic illness. If the sexual appears, it is disclosed because it is present in some form or other in every case of nervous illness, since no nervous illness can take place with a perfectly normal sexual life. The sexual aspect of a neurotic's life is just as important as any other aspect. It is not sexuality which injures the hysteric, it is the over moral repression of it. If the theory of the sexual origin of the neuroses hangs a sword over the head of the hysteric as claimed by some critics, so does the easily proven syphilitic origin of tabes hang a sword over the head of the tabetic.

The problem of sexuality in the neuroses is but one aspect of the problem of the manifestation and distribution of that energy called the libido. This libido is at the very basis of life and of mental conflicts, at first nutritional or self-preservational, and in the second place, the sexual libido or race perpetuation. The word " sexual " is used in a very broad manner in the science of psychoanalysis, in fact, it has the same broad meaning as the word " love." This fact must never be lost sight of in psychoanalysis, since the use of the word by psychoanalysts has been the source of many misconceptions. In primitive tribes, it has also been demonstrated that hysterical attacks may be motivated by an ungratified or a partially gratified erotic feeling.

Q. Is sexual trauma the real cause of a neurosis ?

A. No, because there is scarcely a human being who has not had some sexual shock and yet only a small percentage of people develop a neurosis. If sexual shock were therefore, the cause of a nervous illness, such illnesses would be much more frequent. Besides, many of the stories of sexual shocks which neurotics relate, are found on careful examination to be mere fantastic creations and to have never really taken place. Consequently, during the history of the development of psychoanalysis, the sexual traumatic theory was soon abandoned. It is now evident that the neuroses are due to childhood sexual perversities, the building up of unhealty sexual fantasies and to what is termed the fixation of the neurotic's libido upon his infantile past. This is the real secret of the neurosis, viz. : fantasies which have their root in early childhood and which attach themselves to some one of the family group, usually the father or mother, according to the sex of the subject. It is not the existence of sexual complexes, but their abnormal fixation and over-repression which makes the neurotic.

Q. Since we all have sexual fantasies and repressions, why do some escape a neurosis and some not ?

A. It all depends on the subject's manner of handling his inner life, as to whether he should shut in his personality and become introverted and the victim of wish-fulfilling fantasies (autistic thinking), or whether he becomes active, social, and projects his inner life on healthy activities, that is, extroverted.

Q. What are the deviations of the normal sexual instinct ?

A. These are abnormal sexual manifestations, such as homosexuality or deviations of the sexual object and deviations in regard to the sexual aim, such as attaching an abnormal sexual over-valuation to inanimate objects (fetichism) or the relations between sexuality and pain (sadism and masochism). In the unconscious mental life of many neurotics, can be found deviations from the normal sexual instinct, particularly the Œdipus-complex. It appears that the neurotics are incapacitated by the same unconscious sexual complexes with which the healthy successfully struggle.

Q. What can psychoanalysis do for the sexual hygiene of children ?

A. The proper manner of training the sexual feelings of children, is not to allow these feelings to run rampant. The children should be taught to attach and transfer their instincts to the higher aims of the emotions and intellect, that is, sublimation. Such education should be individual, the instinct should be trained and led. The overcoming of morbid day-dreaming or of abnormal shyness or of an excess of self-admiration (the so-called narcisstic tendency) can do much for the prevention of a later neurosis, since these are unhealthy instinctive reactions fraught with danger.

Q. How is consciousness divided ?

A. Into the foreconscious and the unconscious.

Q What is meant by the foreconscious ?

A. Between the realm of the unconscious and that of consciousness, lies the foreconscious, which contains the material of recent experiences. The foreconscious is therefore that part of consciousness just outside the focus of attention, but which can be easily brought to attention.

Q. What is meant by the unconscious ?

A. The unconscious is that portion of consciousness of which we are not aware.

It is the realm of repressed desires and its material consists of repressed desires and wishes often carried over from early childhood or even infancy. It is a concept or a working hypothesis by which certain mental facts can be controlled, like the ether of the physicists. The unconscious mental life is no more a contradiction in terms of psychology, than certain terms such as "solid solutions" or "invisible light" are in physics. It is to be preferred to the term subconscious, because the latter connotes a spatial relationship. The unconscious is the most important concept of recent times in the realm of mental medicine. It is our historical past and as such, in it is preserved the primitive traits, emotions, and desires of our prehistoric ancestors. The only function of the unconscious is wishing or desiring. In the unconscious are stored wishes and desires, often unethical, which are impossible of fulfilment in reality, because of the action of the censor of consciousness. These wishes are fulfilled in dreams when the censor is weak or absent and allows the unconscious wishes to slip through in the form of a dream.

Q. What is meant by the censor ?

A. The force which represses unwelcome and unpleasant thoughts, for convenience is termed the censor. It is really a defence of the mind against distressing dreams and painful thoughts. It is the censor which prevents unconscious thoughts from becoming conscious.

Q. How does the unconscious manifest itself ?

A. In dreams, in symptomatic actions like slips of the tongue or pen, neuroses and certain mental diseases not of organic origin.

Q. Can a person know his own unconscious ?

A. Only through his dreams, and then not completely so, since the self analysis of dreams can bring up certain resistances, hence for the time being blocking all further thoughts. Many dreams are symbolic and distorted, and the symbols and distortions are unrecognised by the dreamer.

Q. What is symbolism ?

A. This is a term used in psychoanalysis to express the manner of unconscious thinking in a form in which it would be unrecognised by consciousness. A dream is often symbolic, so is often a nervous symptom, when they are expressions of hidden and forbidden wishes repressed in the unconscious. Nervous symptoms are masks behind which a person takes refuge. The symbol is chosen either from the mental content of the individual or it may have a racial or a social basis. In unconscious thinking, the symbols are often used to express sexual concepts, which for moral or ethical purposes cannot be expressed literally. The sexual symbols of neurotic patients are therefore efforts to escape from their attachment to the more grossly sexual. Symbols are not invented, they are only discovered. The symbol is not an arbitrary choice, but has its source in the unconscious, either of the individual or of the race. Hence the close resemblance between dreams and myths, since the myth is the unconscious symbolic expression of the race, and the dream the unconscious symbol of the individual. Symbolism has its origin in the remotest ages of the past. The symbolism of dreams draws its material from this remote ancestry, showing how often the dream is merely a fragment of the mental life of our prehistoric ancestors.

Q. What is the usual history of a patient's efforts to get well before psychoanalysis is tried ?

A. There is usually a history of treatments with tonics and sedatives, the rest cure and the searching after an organic cause for the neurosis. In some cases suggestion or persuasion has been attempted. In the carefully recorded histories of nervous patients it will be found that all these methods have failed because they did not reach the cause of the trouble : they attempted to cure symptoms without any effort to ascertain the origin of the symptoms.

Q. If a person could not have a complete psychoanalysis, but merely told the details of his neurosis to the physician, what sort of advice ought the analyst to give such a person as to the means of making himself most comfortable ?

A. The advice would depend upon the nature of the neurosis, the mental attitude of the patient and the actual conflicts which had arisen. As a rule the attitude of non-resistance is the best advice, since fighting the neurosis or attempting to put a morbid fear or compulsive thinking out of the mind, is likely to render the nervous illness more severe, or at the most, nothing is gained.

Q. What is a mental conflict ?

A. A mental conflict is a battle between two opposing groups of ideas, part of which are acceptable to the patient and part antagonised by the patient. These groups of ideas may be either conscious or unconscious. As a rule conflicts are of a moral nature and frequently refer to the grossly sexual character of the patient's thoughts. The attempt to banish these thoughts produces the conflict and the neurosis. Mental dissociation is the result of conflicts. In every mental conflict there are two opposing forces, the positive or the force of reality, by which we come into touch with the external world, and a negative, through which reality is opposed by shutting off the external world. It is this last which produces the shut-in personality or the negativism which is so characteristic of dementia præcox.

Q. What is dissociation ?

A. Dissociation is the method whereby the mind gets rid of unpleasant or painful repressed complexes. It is really the mind defending itself. In dissociation there is a splitting of the mental processes, so much so, that in cases of obsession or compulsion neurosis for instance, the origin of the compulsive thinking is unknown, since it comes from the unconscious and therefore obtrudes itself as a foreign body in consciousness.

In this splitting of consciousness, the split-off complexes may lead an independent and autonomous existence.

Q. What is the effect of a partial psychoanalysis ?

A. A partial psychoanalysis is like an unfinished surgical operation. It is not radical, it does not cure or even reach the real fundamental difficulty. The surface symptoms are alone removed. Yet a partial psychoanalysis may provide sufficient self knowledge to enable the sufferer to get along more comfortably than if psychoanalysis had not been attempted.

Q. Can a person cure himself of a neurosis by psychoanalytic rules ?

A. No, because his own unconscious is not completely accessible to introspection and furthermore, he will tend to build up his own resistances and yield to them.

Q. Why does psychoanalysis require so much time ?

A. It does not require any more time than the usual methods of sanatorium treatment. It has the advantage over the latter, in that it leaves the patient free to attend to his business or professional interests.

Q. How long does treatment usually take ?

A. This depends upon several factors, that is, the age of the patient, the severity and duration of the neurosis, the managing of the resistances and transferences which occur during the course of the treatment, and finally upon the skill of the psycho-analyst in handling the neurotic material.

Severe neuroses of long duration and with strong resistances may take months to cure, the milder neuroses will frequently recover within a few weeks. Patients should not become discouraged if they do not improve as rapidly as they wish. A slow improvement may be due to unconscious resistances and sufficient time should be given the physician to uncover these resistances and eliminate them.

Q. Why do some patients get better more slowly than others ?

A. Partly because of the nature of the nervous illness, and partly because of the unconscious resistance towards treatment.

Q. What has been the success of psychoanalytic treatment ?

A. Psychoanalysis has been particularly successful in curing those severe forms of

5

nervous illness which have resisted all other forms of treatment. In the sexual neuroses, such as homosexuality, the psychoanalytic method is the only one which offers a hope of cure or even of amelioration of the condition. Early or mild cases of dementia præcox or of mild paranoia, should be given the benefit of psychoanalytic treatment, even if a cure cannot be promised. In the psychoanalytic treatment of stammering, the unconscious difficulties of the speech defect may be greatly ameliorated. The most gratifying results are obtained with cases of hysteria and in the conditions of morbid fears. The compulsion neuroses, that is cases with obsessions, morbid scruples and compulsive thinking, are particularly favourable for psychoanalytic therapy. Psychoanalysis has also helped those cases which show mild depression, and also the non-organic conditions which have been grouped under the name of neurasthenia. The highest percentage of recoveries are in cases of hysteria, morbid fears, compulsion and anxiety neuroses and in homosexuality.

Q. What constitutes a cure with the psychoanalytic treatment ?

A. A nervous illness may be said to be cured if the symptoms disappear and the character of the dreams changes to those experienced by normal individuals. In the anxiety neuroses, the fear should disappear during the day and the anxiety dreams at night. In the compulsion neuroses, recovery may be designated as having taken place, if there are no further compulsive thoughts or acts, and if the calamity dreams disappear.* In homosexuality, there must be a complete disappearance of the homosexual erotic feeling

* See under compulsion neurosis for a definition of calamity dreams.

during the day and of the homosexual dreams at night. A case of dementia præcox can be said to have recovered, if the patient once more comes into complete touch wth reality. To cure a case of hysteria, it is necessary to remove the mental conflict which is at the basis of the hysterical symptoms. The fact that these types of cases can be cured through psychoanalysis, whereas they were unaffected by other therapeutic procedures, is sufficient to invalidate the criticism of those who claim that the case could have been cured without psychoanalysis.

Q. Does psychoanalysis claim invariable successes ?

A. No more than any method of medical treatment claims invariable successes. Failures may be due to lack of transference, poor technique, improperly selected cases, or lack of sufficient time for treatment.

Q. What are the difficulties of psycho-analysis ?

A. The great obstacle in all psycho-analytic treatment is that the patient really does not want to get well. The neurosis acts as a protector from reality, a sort of a shock-absorber from the buffets of life, and thus a conflict arises between the desire to retain the neurosis and the desire to get well. The great fear of every neurotic is the fear that he may lose his neurosis.

Q. What is the effect of psychoanalysis on the neurotic symptoms ?

A. The more recent symptoms disappear first, while the older symptoms are more difficult to remove. As a rule, during the course of a psychoanalysis, there is no further development of new symptoms or at the most, only transitory new symptoms develop, which are of the nature of defence reactions to retain the neurosis. In homosexuality for instance, the depression and anxiety disappear early in the treatment, whereas the more fundamental and deeply seated symptom of the sexual inversion, is more difficult to deal with and is the last to disappear. The character of the dreams changes, they become more symbolised and spiritualised and less grossly sexual during the course of a successful treatment. The primitive unconscious tendencies become less in evidence, in other words, the analysis raises the unconscious to a higher cultural level, it refines and sublimates it. This is the educational influence of psycho-analysis on an individual. The reserve energy is loosened from the neurotic struggles and becomes free for constructive living and social aims. If the nervous symptoms grow worse during the course of the analysis, this must be interpreted as due either to the resistance or to the course of the disease and not to the treatment.

Q. What is meant by sublimation and what bearing does it have on recovery ?

A. The term " sublimation " was first introduced by Freud and was borrowed from the terminology of chemistry. Literally, it means the act of refining and purifying or freeing from baser qualities. The process of sublimation in psychoanalysis is an unconscious one, that is, it takes place without the subject's knowledge. It is the end result of psychoanalysis, since no patient can be said to have been cured, until he has successfully sublimated. Sublimation may be defined as that unconscious conducting of the repressed emotions to a higher, less objectionable and more useful goal. It can occur only when the libido, through psychoanalysis, has been dissociated from the patient's intellectual processes. Therefore, when a patient fights his neurosis or when resistance occurs, sublimation becomes difficult, because the energy is utilised for unpractical purposes. Sublimation is the capacity for replacement or exchange of the original (repressed) aim for a secondary social, religious, scientific or artistic aim. It is really a transference of basic instincts to other interests.

Q. How can one best sublimate ?

A. Sublimation is more or less of an unconscious process, but it can be hastened by assuming a passive attitude towards the neurosis, and so utilising the energy which was formerly wasted in fighting the nervous illness for a more useful purpose. Particular attention should be paid to the religious tendencies of the patient during a psychoanalysis, as some of the most effective sublimations have been along religious lines.

Q. What is done next after the patient is made aware of his buried mental processes ?

A. Nothing. The psychoanalytic method is not merely a diagnostic one but is used for the purpose of treatment. When the patient is made aware of the buried mental processes, he is thereby released from those intense infantile fixations which are at the root of the neurosis and, through this release, the energies can be utilised for more useful social activities. Suggestion merely opposes something to the neurosis, while psychoanalysis takes away the power that the morbid mental processes exert over the patient. Psychoanalysis overcomes resistances, so much so that its chief aim is not so much the uncovering of buried or unconscious mental processes or the knowledge of unconscious thoughts, but the overcoming of inner resistances. ·On the force of these inner resistances, whether weak or strong, depends the rapidity by which the nervous symptoms yield to treatment. The patient may become aware of the meaning of the symptoms within a short space of time and yet the symptoms may continue, thus demonstrating that the cure is due to another factor and not entirely to self knowledge. This factor is the effect of the analysis in overcoming the internal resistances.

Q. How is it possible to tell if a patient is cured by psychoanalysis, that the neurosis will not again manifest itself at some critical period or after an emotional upheaval?

A. In the first place the unconscious sources of the neurosis have been removed through psychoanalysis, and in the second place the analysis has taught the proper method of dealing with actual conflicts. The change in the character of the dreams often furnishes significant hints concerning the future nervous health.

Q. What should be the attitude of the psychoanalyst towards the patient?

A. The psychoanalyst must have as clean a mind as a surgeon has clean hands. The attitude of the psychoanalyst should be that of the sympathetic physician, whose only interest is his patient's recovery, and yet at the same time that of the scientist who is watching and recording a laboratory experiment. The psychoanalyst must know his own individual complexes and resistances and must be able to place himself, as it were, in the situation of the unconscious of the neurosis he is analysing.

Q. What should be the mental attitude of the person during a psychoanalysis ?

A. Absolute frankness and sincerity, concealing nothing from the physician.

Q. What has psychoanalysis to offer, in teaching a neurotic to meet his difficulties ?

A. The neurosis has its sources in the unconscious, and it is therefore something that cannot be vanquished by simply fighting it. It also shows that the patient has thoughts or dreams originating in his unconscious, of which he would never be consciously guilty. Therefore in compulsive thinking, where for instance, the compulsive thoughts are of a grossly sexual nature, the patient is not responsible for these disagreeable thoughts, however much his mind may be bombarded by them even when he is thinking of something else. This latter fact alone shows that they have their origin outside of conscious thinking.

Q. Can psychoanalysis increase the efficiency of a person who has been made inefficient by a nervous illness?

A. Yes, by training the patient to direct his energy to more useful ends than struggling with his neurosis or consuming his energy on his morbid ideas.

Q. What does psychoanalysis teach concerning the mental attitude of a person toward his neurosis ?

A. The first rule is non-resistance, the second that the psychoanalysis takes the responsibility of the mental conflicts of the nervous sufferer.

Q. What rules of mental hygiene does the psychoanalytic theory teach ?

A. That a person must not fight his neurosis when the neurosis takes the form of fears, doubts, compulsive thinking, etc., since fighting makes the neurosis worse. The attitude to be adopted is one of passivity and non-resistance. Mental discipline merely suppresses the feelings and this suppression is like putting the lid down on a

Jack-in-the box.   When the lid is down, the Jack is out of sight, but he is curled up and condensed and ready to spring out again with full force the moment the pressure of the lid (discipline) is removed.   What a neurotic needs is sublimation, and a final sublimation must be emotional rather than intellectual.   Psychoanalysis solves the difficulties of the inner life.   The unconscious self is the real self which will triumph in the final sublimation.   The intense love and hate of neurotics and their constant cravings for sympathy are forms of transference and consequently symptoms of the nervous illness.   Such manifestations should not be ridiculed but should be taken seriously and attempts made to determine their unconscious sources.

Q. Is the advice to " dismiss it from your mind, " sound advice to give to nervous patients ?

A. No. The physician must be interested in the nervous symptoms, he must take it for granted that they belong to the patient's life history, and therefore have a definite meaning or setting in the mental life. The patient cannot ignore his nervous symptoms, his fears or his obsessions, or dismiss them from his mind, any more than he can ignore or dismiss severe pain of organic origin. The advice not to worry or to fight the unpleasant ideas or nervous symptoms, is based upon ignorance or misconception of the fundamental nature and motives of a nervous illness. To advise travel or distractions in amusement is likewise unavailing, because this kind of advice presupposes that the nervous illness is a senseless grouping of complaints, whereas it is really bound up with the sufferer's wishes and mental conflicts, and bears an intimate relation to the life experiences. Explanation and advice however can be made more rational and helpful if based upon psychoanalytic principles.

Q. What should be the attitude of psychoanalysis to the actual conflicts and difficulties of life ?

A. There are many external problems in life which psychoanalysis cannot adjust, but it can adjust the mental attitude towards these problems. These actual conflicts and problems are those of worry, dilemmas, disillusionment, etc. Psychoanalysis cannot actually eliminate these difficulties, but if the real cause of the conflicts is discovered, the mental readaptation often follows spontaneously. With an analysis, the real solution of the problems becomes clear and the former resistance to readjustment overcome. Psychoanalysis points out the solutions from within the mind. Simple advice, based upon what psychoanalysis has revealed to both the patient and physician, can often be very helpful. Psychoanalysis is often a salvation for an existence cramped and difficult to live.

Q. Ought all life worries be psycho-analysed ?

A. To a certain extent, yes, since many worries are attributed to sources from which they do not actually spring, and a brief psychoanalysis may help to clear up the real situation and furnish better insight into the difficulty.

Q. How can psychoanalytic facts be applied to the prevention of the neuroses ?

A. The frequency of nervous diseases is due, not so much to the rush of civilisation as has been so often claimed, but to the injurious overmoral repression of the libido or to the prevailing erroneous ideas concerning sexual morality. The instincts should be conquered through sublimation and not through repression. The science of psychoanalysis is able to penetrate into the unconscious sources of this repression, in both the neurotic and in various types of normal men and women. It is able to point out the path for the utilisation of the repressed energy into sublimation. Marriage is not a panacea for nervousness, since many married men and women become nervous and over anxious in their attitude towards the struggles and problems of life.

The real prevention of the neuroses must come through individual analyses and not through any general propaganda along the lines of mental hygiene, since the latter at its best can only indicate collective rules which cannot be adapted to the complexities of individual minds. It is through the personal efforts of parents, educators, clergymen and also along the lines of sound medical advice given to the developing child, that neurotic disturbances can be prevented. The only or favourite child is particularly liable to be spoiled by parental overaffection, thus leading to an attitude of self-love and self-indulgence, which furnishes the basis for many nervous and mental disturbances of puberty and adolescence.

Q. What is the value of psychoanalysis in explaining character formation ?

A. The unconscious is that region of the mind where the very springs of character take their source and which shape the fundamental features of the character of an individual. Each individual determines his own character and destiny. The characterological traits of a person are not inherited. The character of a person springs deep from his unconsciousness and is made up either of his original childhood impulses and experiences, sublimations of these or reactions against these. For instance, a timid person might by a sort of compensation become aggressive, a spoiled child who has had everything done at his bidding might develop into an impatient adult. A day dreaming child might become taciturn or even shut-in in his tendencies, or a child with too great self-love can never fall in love later, or if he does so, it is transitory and might lead to social difficulties. All character formation has an emotional rather than an intellectual origin. Psychoanalysis is able to penetrate to the origin of certain character traits, and thus be helpful in eliminating characteristics which may be harmful to the individual.

Q. What is a shut-in personality ?

A. This refers to a peculiar mental make-up out of which cases of dementia præcox frequently develop. It is characterised by a tendency to be anti-social, to live a life of reveries, and by a disinclination to come into touch with reality. This is an unhealthy mental attitude, and should be strictly combatted if it once appears in a child.

Q. What is meant by the feeling of inferiority ?

A. This is a concept introduced to explain the make-up of a neurotic individual. Fundamentally nervous people are those who possess the feeling of inferiority to a greater or less extent, such as timidity, lack of courage or self-confidence. Such types of people attempt to compensate for these feelings of inferiority (in the same way that a weak heart will compensate), and thus lay undue stress upon their defective traits, in order to fortify and strengthen them, the coward for instance becoming superlatively brave. This latter mental adjustment is really a form of sublimation, an attempt to conceal the weak points of the personality.

Q. Can psychoanalysis help to eliminate character traits which are detrimental to the individual ?

A. It can to a certain extent, particularly after the mechanism of the character formation has been thoroughly revealed. Analysis often shows that character traits of a detrimental nature may be due to feelings of inferiority, to attempt at repression or overcompensation, or may arise to cover certain trends for the purpose of concealment. The analysis of character is very complex and its traits have a deep root in the unconscious. This shows that character is not a matter of will power but of handling one's inner repressions and the reactions against these. Thus a character trait like a nervous symptom, may be all out of proportion to the underlying unconscious source.

Q. How is the term " wish " used in psychoanalysis ?

A. The term " wish " is used in a very broad sense in psychoanalysis, as indicating all desires, yearnings and ambitions. It is a dynamic concept, which furnishes the working basis for dreams, neurotic symptoms, slips of the tongue, mental conflicts, and the like.

Q. What is the psychoanalytic theory of dreams ?

A. The dream is the true language of the unconscious, its means of expression, although not its only means of expression. A dream is always the fulfilment of a wish, although that wish may not be clear in the dream as remembered. The dream as remembered is termed the manifest content. The wish is concealed in the underlying thoughts which produce the dream. These underlying thoughts are termed the latent content. Every dream has a deep, personal significance for the dreamer, although a dream may be thrown into activity by apparently insignificant thoughts or incidents during the day (dream instigators). The latent content of the dream, which contains the dream wish, may become so distorted and symbolised, that the real origin of the dream may be unrecognised in the manifest content. Occurrences during the day or things read, do not cause the dream, they merely throw the latent or unconscious thoughts into activity.

Q. How is a dream made ?

A. A dream is made by the large mass of latent thoughts of the dreamer becoming condensed into the momentary dream as it is remembered on awakening. We are aware only of the manifest dream: the latent dream thoughts can only be known through an analysis of the dream.

Q. What is the psychoanalytic interpretation of forgetting ?

A. The forgetting of various places and things with which one is familiar is not caused by a mere deterioration of memory, but is an active repression, a purposeful exclusion of the memory from consciousness.

Q. Why do we forget dreams so easily ?

A. The forgetting is a purposeful act. The dream is " forgotten " because it deals with unpleasant material and there is a wish to forget it. The forgetting of a dream is not due to our treacherous memories, but is really a form of resistance. For instance, often in the recital of a dream, a "forgotten portion" is suddenly remembered and this fragment is usually the most important part of the dream.

Q. Does a dream as remembered, always mean what it says?

A. No, because the dream as remembered may be highly condensed or symbolised, or so distorted as to give an opposite meaning to what the dream really connotes. The underlying dream thoughts which produce the dream, conceal the dream wish. The meaning of the dream is hidden in these underlying dream thoughts.

Q. Are all dreams wish fulfilments?

A. Every dream is the fulfilment of a wish. The wish may not be clear in the dream as remembered, yet it can always be found through a psychoanalysis in the latent content of the dream. In dreams of children the wish in the dream is more clearly indicated than in the dreams of adults. In adults the wish is in the latent content and not in the manifest content of the dream.

Q. From what source do the wishes in the dreams originate ?

A. 1. Wishes that arise during the day, but are unfulfilled and so are fulfilled in the dream, such as dreams of children, who frequently dream of dainties or play activities denied them during the day.

2. The wish may come up during the day but may be rejected and repressed, such as feelings of hatred or desires for revenge. These wishes are then completely fulfilled only in the dream, because the ethical fulfilment is impossible in reality.

3. Wishes or desires may arise during the night while sleeping, such as thirst and a wish for water. These wishes are usually fulfilled by a dream of drinking, in order to prevent the sleeping subject from awakening.

4. Wishes deeply buried in the unconscious and carried over from early childhood. This explains why we so often dream of injuring those relatives who are near and dear to us.

Q. Is the wish fulfilment always clear in the dream ?

A. No, because the wish may be highly disguised or distorted and can only be determined through an analysis of the dream.

Q. How is the fact explained that we sometimes dream of the death of one of our

parents, whom we certainly do not consciously wish dead ?

A. It means that the wish existed at one
time in very early childhood and for ethical
reasons was repressed. The meaning of
death to a child has a different connotation
from death to an adult, since the former
denotes merely a removal for the time
being.

Q. What is the function of dreaming ?

A. To protect sleep from the mass of
latent thoughts by making these thoughts
momentary aud unrecognisable by the
sleeper. The only type of a dream which
disturbs sleep is a nightmare.

Q. What is a nightmare ?

A. A nightmare is an anxiety dream.

An anxiety dream is very difficult to explain, since the element of fear in such a dream seems to contradict the theory of wish fulfilment and protection of sleep. This contradiction is more apparent than real however. An anxiety dream means that we have suppressed the desire for certain forbidden pleasures in the unconscious. The suppression produces conflict and pain, the pleasure is throttled and when it escapes it assumes the character of the suppressed pain.

Q. What is the place of the dream in psychoanalysis ?

A. Dream analysis can show a man's latent possibilities and his real ambitions and desires. It portrays the psychological situation of the unconscious and hence dream analysis is an absolute necessity in psychoanalysis. Dream analysis can never become mechanical, although it is based on certain technical rules.

Q. How do the dreams bring out certain things, such as concealed facts unknown to the dreamer?

A. A dream is the product of the unconscious, consequently a dream is an index of unconscious thinking. The free associations of the various elements of dreams furnish the material out of which the dream is made. Much of this material consists of repressed desires which are unknown to the dreamer until the dream analysis has been made.

Q. How does dream analysis help the patient?

A. Through the dreams, the analysis is able to determine the unconscious desires and wishes, the conflicts, transferences and various resistances of the patient. It gives an insight into the unconscious mental life, and thus unravels the mechanism of the neurosis and the repressed material out of which the neurosis is constructed. Sometimes one dream will be found to contain the secret of the neurosis. An elaborate dream is often of less value than a short one, since the latter often reaches to unconscious levels in which lie the very roots of the neurosis. The first dream of the analysis is very important, although in many cases the most difficult to analyse completely, since it often contains the entire mental attitude towards the psychoanalytic procedure. The same theme may appear with many variations and symbols in different dreams.

Q. What is the practical value of dream analysis ?

A. It gives an insight into the unconscious mental life of individuals and of social groups and thus helps in determining the real motives of men and women and of society in general. It has also thrown light on comparative mythology and shown that the psychological structure of a myth is the same as that of a dream. Dream analysis also helps in determining the wishes, resistances, mental conflicts, and jealousies of normal individuals.

Q. If a person does not dream, how is it possible to penetrate the unconscious?

A. Every one dreams, although in some persons the resistance is so great that the dreams are speedily forgotten on awakening. If there is an absolute insistence that no dreams took place, then it is necessary to watch the symptomatic actions or even to utilise artificial dreams, for the penetration of the unconscious.

7

Q. What is an artificial dream ?

A. This is a dream which a person consciously makes up when requested to fabri-
cate what he would consider to be a genuine
dream. Artificial dreams contain the same
distorting mechanisms and have the same
unconscious mental processes as genuine
dreams.

Q. What is meant by typical dreams ?

A. Such dreams as of being insufficiently
clothed, flying, of the death of a near and
dear relative, such as a parent. They are
called typical dreams because nearly every
one has dreamed of them in much the same
manner. The inner meaning of such dreams
arises from emotions which are common to
the entire human race. They consequently
have the same significance in the case of
every dreamer.

Q. Can a dream be interpreted arbitrarily ?

A. Only certain typical dreams can be so interpreted and then only in a superficial manner. A complete dream interpretation requires active co-operation and a knowledge of the person's life interests.

Q. Can every dream be interpreted and analysed ?

A. No, because in some dreams the resistance is so strong and the material out of which the dream is woven lies in such deep strata of the unconscious, that a complete analysis is impossible. This difficulty is due to the fact that the inner resistances interfere with the free associations which are necessary for the analysis of the dream. If these resistances can be overcome, the dream can then be analysed, for instance, it often occurs during the course of psycho-analytic treatment, that a dream which it was impossible to analyse early in the treatment, becomes easily interpreted later.

Q. Can a person analyse his own dreams ?

A. Only to a certain extent, and then only simple wish dreams, typical dreams or those in which the symbols are distinct. In self-analysis of dreams, the interpretation usually given is one desired and not the real analysis, since the resistance prevents an insight into the actual meaning of the dream.

Q. Can dream interpretation also be applied to the workings of normal minds ?

A. Yes, since the dreams of normal individuals often show their repressed wishes, desires, ambitions, jealousies and mental conflicts.

Q. Does heredity have anything to do with a neurosis ?

A. Not directly, only in the sense of an hereditary predisposition. A neurosis is neither inherited nor transmitted, but arises solely from the emotional conflicts of an individual. If we were satisfied with pigeonholing the neuroses as hereditary, it would have barred the investigation of the cause of the neuroses and stopped all efforts at treatment. A neurosis is an acquired characteristic and such a character cannot be inherited. What is so often called heredity in children is merely imitation of their elders.

Q. Why is it that a nervous illness seems to break out suddenly at some critical emotional period ?

A. Because a new adaptation, a kind of a new mental adjustment, becomes suddenly necessary. Then the neurosis breaks out, not because of an emotional shock or from fatigue, but from the emotional trends which the patient for years has repressed in his unconscious. In other words, the neurotic has suddenly become the victim of a regression or return to his infantile fixations. The fatigue or emotional upheaval or anxiety which often precedes such a nervous breakdown, is not its actual cause, but merely its instigator. We are all in danger of a neurosis to a limited degree, because when new difficulties arise, we tend to minimise them by retiring within ourselves. In this mental attitude, difficulties are temporarily removed, but the attitude itself constitutes the neurosis. In other words, a neurosis means that the patient wishes to avoid some task or get away from some new problem of adaptation.

Q. What is the feeling of unreality ?

A. This feeling of the surroundings appearing unreal is a very frequent symptom of many forms of nervous illness. Its origin is very complex. Briefly, it arises because the subject finds reality too painful to bear, and he prefers to live in a world of his own ideas rather than in the world of physical reality. This dominating by the unreality feeling is an unconscious mental process rather than a conscious and deliberate act. It is a condition which can be greatly helped and in many cases cured by psychoanalysis.

Q. Can overwork produce a nervous illness ?

A. Overwork can never produce a neurosis unless the soil has already been prepared for it. Overwork merely reduces the resistance, enabling the neurosis to make its appearance. It does not produce the neurosis because the symptoms are all out of proportion to the actual physical fatigue which antedated the so-called "break-down." Furthermore, the fatigue of which so many nervous patients complain, is false fatigue and not a genuine physical fatigue. For this reason, such patients feel more tired in the morning and the fatigue actually wears off during the day's activities and this also explains why such patients fail to improve with rest.

Q. What is a nervous breakdown from a psychoanalytic standpoint ?

A. Neurasthenia or a nervous breakdown cannot be explained on a purely organic basis. The neurasthenic condition really consists of unconscious desires striving for expression. Many so-called "nervous breakdowns" are really cases of mild periodic depression or of various psycho-neuroses.

Q. What can psychoanalysis do for these nervous breakdowns ?

A. In many cases it can prevent the recurrence of a periodic nervous breakdown by eliminating its unconscious sources or the breakdown may be cured through psycho-analysis.

Q. Is it necessary to dig into and unravel all the fantasies which have become repressed in the patient's unconscious ?

A. Yes, because the energy which the patient needs for the restoration to and the maintenance of his mental health, is attached to these repressed fantasies. By dragging the fantasies into consciousness they become detached from the libido and the reserve energy of the patient can then be utilised to more useful ends, or in technical terms, become sublimated. Thus psychoanalysis helps the patient to adequately meet the tasks of life, and in a moral sense it re-educates and reconstructs him. The real cure in psychoanalysis comes from within, for after all the conscious material has been thoroughly considered, the dreams are next investigated, as these furnish the unconscious material which is producing the neurosis.

Q. What is hysteria ?

A. Hysteria is due to ideas which are out of harmony with the rest of the personality. These ideas are repressed and this repression is at the basis of all hysterical manifestations. It is the repression which causes the dissociation of hysteria. The repressed ideas may be converted into the peculiar

mental states and conditions of forgetful-
ness (amnesia) of hysteria or they may be
converted into the physical symptoms of
hysteria, such as paralysis, blindness, losses
of sensation, feelings of unreality, etc.
Hysteria is, therefore, the effort of the
human mind to disguise its unpleasant
thoughts and experiences, and as such,
hysteria always represents a mental conflict.

Q. What is anxiety hysteria ?

A. This is a form of nervous disease
which is associated with various morbid
fears. With these fears there is associated
the usual psychological accompaniments of
the emotion of fear, such as difficulty of
breathing, palpitation of the heart, trem-
bling and sometimes disturbances of the
stomach and intestines. Many so-called
nervous children are sufferers from anxiety
hysteria.

Q. What is an anxiety neurosis ?

A. This is sometimes difficult to distinguish from anxiety hysteria. Many cases of stammering, and so-called neurasthenia are really cases of an anxiety neurosis.

Q. What is the psychoanalytic theory of stammering, and what can psychoanalysis do for the treatment of stammering ?

A. Stammering is a form of an anxiety neurosis. The motivating mechanism which causes stammering is unknown to the sufferer, that is, it is unconscious, the only conscious reaction being that of anxiety, fear, and difficulty of talking. The distributing element in stammering is mental and not physical, it is more than a mere affection of speech. The attempt to repress from consciousness into the unconscious certain trends of thought or emotions is the chief mechanism in stammering. The repressed thoughts, because of fear of betrayal, come into conflict with the wish to speak and not to betray, and hence the stammering arises. The cure for stammering can be attained only through an exploration of the unconscious, and a complete breaking down of those resistances which in early childhood produced the stammering. Phonetic or speech training can accomplish but little or at the most can produce only temporary results in stammering. It is necessary to know all the stammerer's fears and their origin before sound advice can be given concerning the mental attitude towards the difficulties of talking.

Q. What is a compulsion neurosis?

A. Cases with compulsive thinking, such as obsessions and doubts, constitute a compulsion neurosis. It was formerly termed psychasthenia. A compulsion neurosis is a very complex disturbance, and its ramifications in the mental life are deep and far reaching. Its mechanism is probably a transferred self-reproach from something which has been repressed into the unconscious. This is particularly shown by the frequent appearance of what may be termed "calamity dreams." These are types of dreams in which harm or evil appears to be happening to others. Such wishes are strongly repressed in the unconscious and consequently are only revealed in the dream.

Q. What is the psychoanalytic interpretation of kleptomania?

A. In a case of kleptomania, if feeblemindedness and actual insanity can be eliminated, the kleptomania is very likely a form of a compulsion neurosis.

Q. What is psychoanalysis able to do for cases of maniac depressive insanity ?

A. It can be very helpful. Many of the mild cases of manic-depressive insanity, which are termed cyclothemia, are in reality cases of anxiety hysteria. Their only resemblance to the manic-depressive group is in their periodicity. Many cases of depression and even of exaltation, will be found on analysis to be the patient's method of getting away from reality or in reaction to unconscious emotional strain. The depression and excitement arise from mental conflicts. The depression is an overwhelming of the mind by repressed emotions, the excitement is an effort to keep the painful ideas out of the mind. Many cases of periodic neurasthenia or mild periodic depression can be distinctly helped or even absolutely cured through the analytic investigation of the underlying cause of the mental disturbance, since many of these cases are really due to a lack of emotional adaptation. Cases with perodic depression often show a constitutional tendency to depressed states, and it is here that psychoanalysis may make a change for the better.

Q. What can psychoanalysis do for alcoholism ?

A. Provided there are no evidences of alcoholic mental deterioration, psycho-analysis can help, and in many instances cure, cases of periodic alcoholism. The drinking habit is due to complex mental factors, which are merely instigated by temptation and opportunity. The real underlying cause of a sudden alcoholic bout is unknown to the sufferer. Psychoanalysis is often able to determine the cause and thus remove it. In many cases, periodic alcoholism is due either to an effort to get away from reality or in reaction to suppressed sexual desires. The impelling cause of many cases of alcoholic indulgence, or the compulsive, irresistible feeling to drink, lies in the unconscious.

Q. Is it possible to help a case of dementia præcox by psychoanalysis?

A. Only early, mild or latent cases of dementia præcox are suitable for psychoanalytic treatment. Even if it is impossible to cure a case of dementia præcox, many of the symptoms may be largely relieved. Furthermore, a psychoanalytic investigation of a dementia præcox patient will often furnish information concerning the problem of regulating the life interests. Dementia præcox may be interpreted as a functional mental disturbance, a form of dissociation of the personality, with a withdrawal of personal interests from reality in much the

8

same way as hysteria, but of a more intense form.

Q. How does the usual medical history of a nervous illness differ from a psychoanalysis ?

A. The usual accounts given by patients of their nervous illness do not reproduce the entire story, no matter how honest the individual may be in his attempt to relate all the facts, or how keen the memory in stating the details. Under these conditions only the superficial data are given, since consciousness conveniently " forgets " those incidents which are disagreeable to the personality and represses these into the unconscious. These repressed memories can be withdrawn from the unconscious only by the work of psychoanalysis.

Q. What is the ethical value of psychoanalysis ?

A. Psychoanalysis teaches that the unconscious gets its gratification through a symbolic outlet, either in the form of dreams or of neurotic symptoms. Repression is the most important factor in our civilised life. It keeps individuals from doing harm even if they have evil thoughts. The repressed feelings however are not lost ; there is no waste of energy, since these feelings are sublimated or utilised for a higher and more useful purpose. Psychoanalysis encourages a more honest form of thinking, both in individuals and in social groups. It gives an insight into the real workings of our minds and our feelings and teaches us what we really are. There is a constant tendency in all of us to a self-deception : we conceal our real thoughts and feelings through illogical deductions or in obedience to what we term moral conduct. This process is termed rationalisation. Psychoanalysis penetrates into the unconscious motives of our thoughts and actions, and shows, how without self-deception, we can best utilise our inner feelings for the conduct of life.

Q. What bearing has psychoanalysis on education ?

A. The purpose of psychoanalysis is to utilise the energy of an individual so that it will find a natural outlet. As such, psycho-analysis is educational in its scope, since it tends to utilise for practical purposes all that is best in an individual. The earliest years of childhood are very important for good health and sound character, and it is in these early years that education based on psychoanalytic principles is most effective for the prevention of a future nervous illness or the formation of undesirable character traits. Many of the bad habits of children, such as lying or stealing, may be early forms of a future compulsion neurosis. Children should be encouraged to find suitable outlets for their interests, otherwise their interests may be turned inward on themselves, leading to those day-dreams and mental conflicts, which so often produce a neurosis. Particularly to be avoided is the impressing of children with feelings of guilt, shame or terror, by insistence on punishment, or frightening the child with bogies.

Q. What is the future of psychoanalysis?

A. The future of psychoanalysis depends upon the improvement in its technique, the general cultural advance of psychoanalytic investigation, careful statistical studies of the effect of the method by different workers in the field and finally making physicians more familiar with the theory and practice of psychoanalysis. It will aid in the prevention of neuroses by giving an insight into the real mechanisms which produce nervous breakdowns, such as, that nervous invalidism is not due to overwork, but to repressed emotions and unsatisfied instincts. The psychoanalytic method of investigating unconscious mental processes is full of promise for the future.

HINTS FOR READING

K. ABRAHAM—*Dreams and Myths*—1913.

A contribution to comparative Mythology showing that the same elements enter into the structure of both dreams and myths.

ALFRED ADLER—*The Neurotic Constitution*—1917.

A psychological analysis of the mental make-up of nervous sufferers.

A. A. BRILL—*Psychoanalysis*—1913.

A series of papers on the theories and the practical application of psychoanalysis.

ISADOR H. CORIAT—*Abnormal Psychology*—1914.

An outline of the entire field of Abnormal Psychology.

The Meaning of Dreams—1915.

A general outline of the meaning of dreams, their relation to the unconscious and the problems of psychoanalysis.

The Hysteria of Lady Macbeth—1912.

A psychoanalytic interpretation of the character of Lady Macbeth.

*Psychoneurosis Among Primitive Tribes—Journal
of Abnormal Psychology—*1915.

A study of hysterical attacks in the primitive men of the Fuegian Archipelago.

S. FERENCZI—*Contributions to Psycho-Analysis*
—1916.

A series of papers dealing in a highly technical manner with various aspects of psychoanalysis.

SIGMUND FREUD—*The. Interpretation of Dreams—*
1914.

The fundamental work on psychoanalysis in which the mechanism of dreams and the functions of the unconscious are discussed in great detail.

*Three Contributions to the Sexual Theory—*1912.

The entire question of sexual development is discussed from a new and broader view-point.

*Leonardo da Vinci—*1916.

A psychoanalytic character study of the great Italian painter.

*Wit and its Relation to the Unconscious—*1916.

A study of the mental process of wit and laughter.

*The Psychopathology of Everyday Life—*1914.

A study of the unconscious actions of normal persons.

The Origin and Development of Psychoanalysis—
1910.

Five Lectures delivered at the Twentieth Anniversary of Clark University, and giving a history of the psychoanalytic movement by its founder.

BERNARD HART—*The Psychology of Insanity* —1912.
A psychoanalytic study of mental diseases.

E. HITSCHMANN—*Freud's Theories of the Neuroses* —1913.
The significance of psychoanalysis for medicine.

EDWIN B. HOLT—*The Freudian Wish*—1915.
The relation of psychoanalysis to ethics with a discussion of the function of the " wish " as a key to the mind.

ERNEST JONES—*Papers on Psychoanalysis*— 1913.
A collection of papers on the applications of psychoanalysis.

C. G. JUNG—*Psychology of the Unconscious*—1916.
A contribution to the history of the evolution of thought on the basis of the analysis of unconscious thinking.

Analytical Psychology—1916.
A collection of papers previously published, on the various therapeutic aspects of psychoanalysis.

OSCAR PFISTER—*The Psychoanalytic Method* —1917.
The application of Psychoanalysis to the education of children.

What is Psychoanalysis?

J. J. PUTNAM—*Human Motives*—1915.

A study of human motives from a psycho-analytic viewpoint.

O. RANK AND H. SACHS—*The Significance of Psychoanalysis for the Mental Sciences*—1916.

A contribution to the cultural aspects of psychoanalysis.

WM. A. WHITE—*Mechanisms of Character Formation* —1916.

Human character interpreted according to psychoanalytic principles.

WILFRID LAY—*Man's Unconscious Conflict*—1918.

A sound popular exposition of Psychoanalysis, by a whole-hearted disciple.

Among journals, may be mentioned the *Psychoanalytic Review*, published quarterly, and *the Journal of Abnormal Pyschology*, published bi-monthly. The former is devoted exclusively to the various medical and cultural aspects of psychoanalysis: the latter contains a large number of psychoanalytic articles.

INDEX

Index